Femdom Temptations

Explore Your Submissive Desires and Transform your Sex life

(five ready-to-use 30-min femdom hypnosis sessions)

Alexandra Morris

Contents

Introduction: Why this book is for you 1

Script One: *You Are Not a Macho Man. Healing the Submissive with Gentle Femdom* 6

Script Two: *Pain or Pleasure, Which Do You Choose?*...........22

Script Three: *Blindfolded with Tied Balls. How Much Can You Handle?*..38

Script Four: *Say Hello to My Little Friend*....................54

Script Five: *Fulfill Your Mistress's Dreams. Say Hi to Her Bull* 69

Erotic Hypnosis Audio Recordings.............................83

Conclusion 84

Connect With Me 89

Introduction: Why this book is for you

Whenever I bring up erotic hypnosis, I tend to get strange looks. I've been told time and time again about how erotic BDSM hypnosis sounds like something that belongs in a dark fantasy romance; however, the results of it speak for themselves. My Erotic Hypnosis books, *"Erotic Hypnosis: A Beginner's Crash Course (Including Femdom,* and *Female-Led Relationships Scripts) and "Erotic Hypnosis: Six Sessions of Guided Femdom Meditation (ready-to-use scripts),"* have already helped countless individuals and couples to find a whole new world of sexual pleasure and erotic self-empowerment. This book is the next boundary-pushing installment in the series.

Skepticism isn't unexpected. After all, new hasn't always had the best reputation, and hypnosis is still not widely considered a legitimate part of psychology, despite proof that it works. Usually, a person's first reaction to the words "erotic hypnosis" is assuming that something sinister and non-consensual may be involved. Hypnosis has often been misrepresented in media as the means to brainwash someone into performing feats they otherwise wouldn't. You might also be worried about things being planted in your subconscious without your consent. This is not the case.

Neither BDSM nor hypnosis seek to take control of you outside of sex play and intercourse. BDSM is an umbrella term for a spectrum of practices that focus on power exchange during sexual intimacy. It can include exhibitionism, voyeurism, pain play, roleplaying, etc., and it can truly help cultivate a healthy sex life.

Even though it remains a taboo, BDSM has been present in cultures around the world for centuries. Just like erotic hypnosis, it might seem extreme or unconventional to an outsider, but it can be a more profound way to explore one's consciousness, control, power, and the fem/masc dynamics in a relationship.

Recent studies on BDSM have revealed astonishing results about its effects. Not only is there no evidence of causing harm, but BDSM might even positively impact physical and mental health, boost the imagination, reduce stress, and deepen relationships.

Experienced BDSM practitioners typically display a high level of communication skills and sex education. The "scenes" usually require a lot of planning and safety precautions, as well as a strong sense of decisiveness, vulnerability, and cooperation. These also happen to be the basis of a healthy and positive relationship.

It's vital to be aware that it is perfectly alright to be submissive in a consensual way, and to understand that submitting sexually does not reflect the relationship dynamics emotionally or the roles outside the realm of sex play.

BDSM can also immerse you in a Zen-like state, that is, the high one gets from intense exercise, making it an excellent companion to erotic hypnosis.

Fundamentally, erotic hypnosis is a tool to help you get in touch with your most secret desires. It can unleash parts of yourself that are hiding between layers of social conditioning and taboos through meditation and theta brainwaves.

Our brains experience several electrical impulses throughout the day, which determine the type of communication that is taking place between our neurons and our brain. The primary five brainwave states are Gamma, Alpha, Beta, Delta, and Theta. Theta waves are the ones we will be using to help you learn how to consciously bridge the gap between your conscious and your subconscious.

The theta state is a fascinating mode that sits right on the edge of both the conscious and the subconscious and lets us pay attention to subtle things that we would otherwise miss. It would be the equivalent of "repair mode" on a computer as we become better at identifying suppressed emotions and areas in our bodies that we're not addressing while conscious.

This is the state that we can explore and exploit to have a lot of fun. We're still just barely aware of our thoughts, so there is potential for a massive flow of ideas and inspirations than when we're in an active, brainstorming mode. This is the reason a lot of people get amazing inspiration and ideas while showering, jogging, or falling asleep. The brain gets into theta state! When triggered, we relax on a much deeper level. Intuition increases while anxiety and stress decline; mental blocks vanish. Our brains also expand to emotions we tend to suppress.

The transition to theta usually just occurs on its own, but you can learn how to trigger it at will!

You should take your time to practice going into theta for about fifteen minutes per day. Inevitably, though, modern rhythms of life tend to get in the way of our well-being, and we often skip attuning to the nuances of our body and mind. Cultivating your ability to slip into theta is not only going to be great for your sexual life, but also excellent for learning how to feel, think, and express yourself more clearly for the rest of your day.

I've written this book for men and couples who are intrigued by femdom, hypnosis, sexual ASMR, and sexual meditation. If you are a man who's been dreaming of living out your most intimate and "taboo" desires and fantasies, this book will give you a chance to do so. It's also an excellent read for women who wish to play the role of the "Mistress" in a femdom-led relationship. It is a book that pushes boundaries and that will be crude, vulgar and lewd at times, as it will dig deep into your deepest desires.

There are five progressive scripts included. While this book serves as a "partner" and a stress-relief, it can also serve as a guide to you if you're a couple who wishes to practice erotic hypnosis at home. You can read them on your own or out loud for your partner, and either practice getting into a meditative state or act out the scripts as roleplay. You could even record them and listen to them afterward. You can, of course, satisfy yourself during the sessions; in fact, it is highly encouraged so you can achieve the greatest degree of pleasure!

Script One

You Are Not a Macho Man. Healing the Submissive with Gentle Femdom

Well, hello there. What have we here? A tough, rugged macho man? **[chuckle]** We shall see about that... I can see you're bursting with anticipation, aren't you? You're curious about how you, a **[gently sarcastic]** tough, rugged, macho man, will interact with someone like me. In this session, we'll address potential emotional and mental blocks that might have been installed in you long ago. It's best if you practice with this session regularly, especially if you feel the prejudices and insecurities begin to rise again. So, shall we get started?

Alright, my darling pet. First, I need you to get very, very comfortable. Moving to a dark and safe space would be ideal. I don't want you to get distracted while listening to my voice.

Do you think you are ready for me? That's cute. You are *so* cute. **[small pause]** What's that? You don't like me calling you cute? Do you think calling you cute makes you sound less manly? How adorable you are! Together we will shed those insecurities. I believe you will feel so much better after that, don't you? But first, let's get you ready.

All right? Have you found your space yet? It's better if it's nice and dark. **[small pause]** Any place that you feel comfortable in is a great choice. You may sit or lie down. If you want, you may even draw a hot, fragrant, relaxing bath and submerge your body in the water. Just get comfortable and close your eyes. **[smaller pause]** Are you ready? Good boy. Are you comfy? Aw, you are such a good *boy*.

I sense that you don't like me calling you "boy." Is it because you think you are a big, manly alpha male? But you're not really that macho, are you, my boy? Allow yourself to relax and explore that hidden inner part of you that knows that you're a gentle, obedient sub. I will help you reach it. You knew what you were getting into when you sought me out, my pet. In reality, all that you desire deep inside is to comply with my will and do my bidding. You cannot wait for me to start so that you can jump into this experience with both feet. You are so eager and pliable, my pet. A compliant, acquiescent, and loyal submissive. Just imagine how wonderful and fun it will be to close your eyes while I take over. Just imagine how wonderful will it be to surrender control, to not have to worry about taking care of everything yourself. Just imagine how lovely and freeing it will be when I finally strip away that macho man mentality, and you can realize your true self and fulfill your deepest fantasies.

Imagine how wonderful you will feel when you are finally liberated from the burden of always being in control. My voice will get you there and free you.

I will help you by admitting that you too have needs, and it is good to pay heed to those needs. I will help you leave all of your limiting views, your stressful ambitions, and your outdated convictions behind. You don't need me to massage your ego. You will leave all of that ego behind and just leave yourself in my hands and my voice and the darkness. I will help you liberate yourself from the insatiable need to be competitive and just focus on your deeper self, your desires, and your needs. I will help you become one with your own desires and feelings. You will just obey my voice. You might feel a twitch right now, trying to make you object that you do not need help. Ignore it. Focus only on the sound of my voice and the shape of my words. It is the only thing you want to listen now. You will submit to my voice, gradually, with each breath.

Now, inhale deeply. In through the nose, and hold while I count.

One. Two. Three. Four. Five.

Now exhale slowly, through your mouth. Don't rush it. Slow and languid. That's it. Good boy.

One more time, inhale deeply through your nose.

One. Two. Three. Four. Five.

Release it again, slowly.

Well done. Keep going.

Deep breath.

One. Two. Three. Four. Five.

And out.

Deep breath.

One. Two. Three. Four. Five.

And out.

Deep breath.

Think of all the social expectations of masculinity that are holding you back.

One. Two. Three. Four. Five.

And let them out.

You are floating on a soft, fluffy, white cloud, naked. The surface under you is becoming softer, like cotton. Feel the mild and pleasant breeze stroking your skin. You take a deep breath. One. Two. Three. Four. Five.

And exhale.

You can feel your lovely cloud rising, wrapping around you. You are surrounded by protective swaths of fluff. The softness of the cloud spreads through your body. You are now beginning to relax.

You are worthy of relaxation because I have chosen you. No need for you to be active all the time. Relax. I know you are very intelligent. I know you feel the urge to react because you want to remain in charge, but I want you to stop acting and reacting now. Just lay back, relax, and let my voice take charge and guide you.

Your cloud now rises a little more. It's taking you up. The room slowly vanishes from around you, and you can now feel warmth. The sun is shining down on you as you drift. You can feel its heat spreading on your chest, down your torso. You can feel your shoulders relax, cradled in the softness of the cloud.

The sun's warmth is coursing through your body, from your torso to your pelvis, down your legs. Your muscles relax. Tension slips out and away like mist. The heat is moving to your toes and your arms, and you relax, feeling loose and free. Floating. Your forehead is nice and warm. Comfortable. Let the warmth spread down to your neck. Inhale. One. Two. Three. Four. Five.

Feel the cloud supporting you. You can let go of the stress of carrying everything and everyone now. The cloud is soft yet sturdy. Notice each part of your body that touches it. It is so comfortable. There is no more stress or pain, no more responsibilities. There is only comfort and warmth.

Feel the cloud beneath. It feels chilly and a little damp, like early morning grass. It feels wonderful. The breeze is keeping you cool. The sun's warmth radiates to your stomach. Feel the warmth spreading inside you, the contrast with the coolness of the cloud.

The cloud is floating higher and higher. You can float wherever you please. You're safe. The sky is blue and calm. Other clouds float past you lazily. It is very relaxing and tranquil. I know you want to stay ever active, but you won't. Laziness now is good. Relax and let your body slip into idleness. You are obedient. You are worthy of laziness, for I have chosen you. You do not need to be rushing about and around.

The sun's warmth is spreading on you like melting butter. It extends down to the bottom of your stomach and along your length, filling it, coursing down to your balls. You are now fully immersed in comfortable warmth. You are secure. You are now fully at peace. Relaxed. Calm. Secure.

The grass seems further and further away as you rise high in the sky. The breeze is getting a little stronger, but it's still mild enough. The warmth within lingers as the breeze keeps you comfortable. You can feel the breeze between your toes, caressing, cooling your feet, while the warmth stays inside you and begins to buzz and tingle through your body.

The horizon is all around you. A lovely circle of blue and sun and warmth. You sway gently like a boat on smooth water. Enjoy the languid rocking of the cloud. Your body begins to tingle at the breeze against your sun-warmed skin.

You can feel the softness and coolness of the cloud on your bottom, and your back relaxing. Your arms and your hands tingle. Your fingers feel the cotton-like smoothness of the cloud. The softness tickles your neck, and it cradles your head. Feel the soft caress against your head, like gentle feathers.

Focus on the feather-like feeling. Let the feathers touch you, kiss you. Submit to the feathers. Every touch releases pleasure; it makes you care for others.

Submit to the feathers. You need the help of the feathers. Have faith in them. Feel the sensation fill your head. Now feel the softness move down your body, through your chest, through your stomach; feel it crossing all the way down to your legs and toes. Feel the touch of the feathers inside like gentle kisses. Feel the breeze swirl around your stomach. Submit to the softness. The pleasure. Submit.

Let your feelings and emotions penetrate you like the sunshine penetrated your body. You don't need to hide your emotions, your fears, and your anxiety now. You are safe here. High in the sky and deep inside you. Inhale and feel the strength of all the emotions you have been suppressing. You are not a macho man. No. You are a loyal, pliant, emotional pet. Good boy.

Exhale and let out all the fear, anxiety, and stress.

You do not need to be in charge anymore. Let my voice guide you. Have faith in my voice.

Allow yourself to feel my voice, soothing you. You can be vulnerable now. Let yourself be entranced by the shape of my words. Feel their vibrations penetrate your thoughts and get you entranced. You are not a macho man. No. You are susceptible and exposed but safe. Vulnerable, but you trust your Mistress.

You have floated up at the highest you can reach, and you feel peaceful and calm, drifting into the vast blue sky. The breeze is cool on your skin, and the sunshine is kissing your insides. Relaxation makes your body tingle with peace. Your fingers and toes tingle softly as you are cradled in the malleable softness of the cloud.

Submit to it. Submit to the sky. The cloud will keep you safe.

The breeze guides you gently further and further. There is only the cloud, the sky, you. Relax on the soft cloud and submit.

The sunshine is my hands. Submit. The breeze is my voice. Submit.

Keep breathing. In through the nose. One. Two. Three. Four. Five.

Out through the mouth.

The cloud embraces you, keeping you safe. My arms embrace you, keeping you safe. The sunshine warms up your soul. My voice warms up your soul. Submit to it.

Your needs are important but pleasing me is more so. You are worthy of pleasing me, for I have chosen you. You are worthy of discarding your insecurities and your conditioning, for I have chosen you. You are worthy of being my submissive, for I have chosen you. You are worthy of being vulnerable, comfortable, and safe, for I have chosen you. Submit. For I have chosen you. Inhale. One. Two. Three. Four. Five. Exhale.

You are worthy of being my submissive.

Say it: You are worthy.

Speak up. You are worthy.

Feel the heat inside you begin to churn and swirl and twist. It moves along the length of your limbs, your torso, slowly and gently along the length of your cock.

You are getting hard. As you're getting harder, your self-importance melts away and becomes confidence. You feel the warmth of the sunshine and the gentle touch of the breeze on your cock.

Feel that warmth that's gathered inside you, filling up your cock. Submit.

My hands are cool on your skin, like the breeze. They touch you and comfort you. Taking control. Caressing everywhere that you wish to be touched. The breeze, my hands that are cool, wrap around your length and pull softly. The breeze becomes my voice. Calling to you. Obey. Submit.

The cloud is soft and comforting, keeping you floating, the breeze is cool and gentle, and sways your body softly. You are hovering between my voice and my hands, and you will obey and submit. You are worthy of letting go. Feel the sweet buzz inside you. Feel the warmth inside you, feel the feathers kissing your skin. They are my kisses. Submit and obey.

You are floating on the cloud. You are cradled in my arms. My hands are gently stroking your cock. Listen to my voice and obey. You *will* submit.

You are vulnerable. You are emotional. You are gentle. You are empathetic. You are worthy. You are submitting.

The breeze is getting warmer. It is my lips and my breath. My lips are right over yours. You feel my hot breath on your face, your lips tickling the soft hairs on your cheeks and your upper lip. You breathe in my breath. My breath floods your body with warmth. You will submit to me.

Your ego shuts down, and you pay attention to my voice and only my voice. Your only real purpose now is to make your Mistress happy. You are submitting.

Feel yourself letting go of all those things that constrict you. Feel all of your learned limitations and behaviors leave your body and mind as you exhale. Relax in my arms and obey the sound of my voice. Submit. Your mind empties of toxic masculinity and fills with submission and obedience.

Now, inhale deeply and hold it as I count.

One. Two. Three. Four. Five.

Once more.

One. Two. Three. Four. Five.

You are vulnerable. You are submissive. You are gentle.

Submit.

Good boy. Feel the tide of acceptance flooding your insides. Sexual desire radiates from you. You want to please your Mistress. Your cock is buzzing and tingling. Your stomach aches with desire as the blood pumps through your veins, ready to fill your cock even more. Ready to please your Mistress. Ready to submit.

Your ego is completely gone. You are worthy of asking for help. I will help you be the best of yourself. Not a macho man. Not an alpha. No. Only a submissive and worthy slave.

Lose yourself in my voice. Lose yourself in the sound of it. Feel your mind and your body submitting fully to what your Mistress needs.

You leave all of your ambitions and convictions behind and feel your desires taking over. You submit to them gradually, with each breath you take. You feel your cock growing larger and larger as you breathe in the energy of the bright blue sky all around you, you feel yourself submitting completely to your desires. You are now drifting, powerless. You don't have any control or say. You only listen to my voice. You are powerless when it comes to your desires. Your cock is buzzing and aching with desire. You become one with your deepest desires. You become one with the need to submit to my voice. Submit.

Hold on to that feeling and picture yourself in your new reality. You are mine now. You are my slave. My loyal slave.

Now, I am no longer talking to the macho man but the obedient slave you know you want to be. I have reached the inner place of your mind, where all of your longing and your desire is deeply seated, bubbling, longing to erupt. Longing to come to the surface. You will stop being in charge now. Your only desire is to submit to me willingly. Let go now. Follow my voice and listen to my every command like a good slave. Doesn't it feel incredible to finally let go and let your Mistress be in control?

Good boy.

Every time you catch yourself thinking you should be in charge, I want you to remember this moment and how good it felt to surrender to my voice and me. Breathe in the change. One. Two. Three. Four. Five. Breathe out and welcome to your new reality as a slave. My slave.

You feel all those lovely sensations from before now culminate into one dominant feeling. You feel like you always were meant to feel. Comforted, malleable, and submissive. You are not an alpha. You are the opposite of an alpha. Your Mistress will take care of you. You can feel that truth rushing through your veins, and it makes your cock grow larger still. You feel invigorated because this truth has set you free. You are a slave as you were meant to be, and it makes you happy. Your Mistress knows your needs and will satisfy every single one of them. You have let go completely and given in to me. All your socially constructed restraints have lifted off and departed so you can align with your truest desires, which is to serve.

The sky is starting to get darker, but you are not cold. You keep the sun's heat inside you, and it keeps you safe and warm. The bright blue is changing to a deeper hue, bursts of pink and gold appearing down below on the horizon as the sun begins its descent. You are peaceful and calm, comfortable in your new reality as a submissive. You are not an alpha. You belong to me. You are my slave.

The sun on the horizon paints the last bits of the lit sky with lovely oranges and golds. The sky above you has darkened completely, and you begin to see little diamond pinpricks like stars. There are thousands of them, and you feel the light of each one like a gentle kiss on your body. You're comfortable and calm and peaceful.

You breathe in the night air, and you let it fill you with a new purpose. That of being not an alpha, but my slave. Focus on this purpose and let it spread through your body. Send it to your genitals and let it fill you. Exhale all of your remaining blocks. You don't need them when your Mistress is around. Inhale the energy from the stars and hold it. Let it spread to your cock, and feel it tingling, growing. Feel the goosebumps from the stars kissing your skin, giving you impossible, unimaginable pleasure and a tiny pinprick of pain. It feels so good, erotic, warm, and delightful. You feel safe and sensual.

Now we will repeat this process. Transfer the energy of the universe and the knowledge that you are my slave to your genitals, and think of nothing else. Inhale deeply, breathing in the energy of the stars. Hold it and make it spread to your stomach and your genitals. It becomes more intense. It becomes so good and erotic and sensual. The process becomes automatic. Every time you breathe, inhaling and exhaling, you can feel the energy and your new reality coming in and spread through your body. You can feel the forces of the universe healing you, taking away toxic ideas and notions, making you pliable like dough. Healing your ego into compassion and empathy. Healing your cockiness into confidence.

Healing your aggression into vulnerability and emotional balance.

Breathe in. You are young and strong. Breathe out. You are healthy and empathetic. Breathe in. You live to please your Mistress. In return, I will satisfy your deepest, most unspeakable desires. Breathe out. You are confident that you are able to please your Mistress. Breathe in. Feel my hands on your length. Breathe out. Feel my lips on your chest. Breathe in. You are safe with me. Breathe out. You can now accept all the aspects of yourself, including that of being my slave and not an alpha. Breathe in. You can now finally accept and respect your needs and acknowledge your desires. Breathe out. The most important of those desires is submitting to your Mistress willingly. Breathe in. The acceptance of your new reality and realizing your sexual fantasy fills you with arousal and joy. Breathe out. You are worthy of pleasing your Mistress.

Good job. You are so good at this, boy. You are now in an elevated state of self-introspection. There is nothing between you and your subconscious. You are extremely suggestible to all of my affirmations. You know that my voice is simply the echo of what you really think.

Continue your breathing and let in more energy. Allow your length to harden. I am right here with you. Feel the goosebumps on your skin. Feel your arousal filling your cock. As you continue to breathe in and out, you feel the path my nails are grazing down your neck, along your torso, down to your length. The path glows and fills you with warmth. It is soft, sensual, comforting. Submitting to me overwhelms you with arousal and well-being.

Good boy, you're learning so fast.

Your cloud now begins its descent. You love the sense of swaying in the night sky with the late evening breeze around you. The sun has set, and there is no moon in the sky, only the stars. You are surrounded by darkness and the magical energy of the universe. You are overcome with sexual euphoria. You know you can always return here, and that this world is as tangible as the one you're accustomed to. I will remain here, waiting for you, and you will obey my every command without a second thought. Feel my lips on your torso, embrace how soft and sensual it feels. The kisses are slowly descending close to your cock. You will remember how fantastic this trance felt. How real, and soft, and sensual, and liberating. This will soon start to feel like your natural state of being. You will be able to tap back into it without any effort at all.

You are relaxed in mind and body. Submitting to me. Devoted to me. Vulnerable to me. Your cock is at full arousal now, and you feel as though it reflects on your entire body. You can feel how hard you are, the energy of the universe pumping in your member like a throbbing heart. You love this pressure and the slight tingle of pain from it. Feel it hum and buzz through your body as my voice only makes it stronger, more energized. You now know how to slip into this trance the next time you hear my voice.

Your cloud is landing on the soft, cool grass. Your arousal has nearly reached its climax. There is precum leaking from your member. Feel how warm it is, dripping down your length, leaving a sultry, erotic path. Good boy.

Your entire body is throbbing, eager for your Mistress and the next time you will meet me. You are such a good slave. When you exit this trance, you will not be an alpha but a sensual, considerate slave. You will be flooded with thoughts of me and being with me throughout your day. You will remember how good and sensual and erotic it felt. You'll be refreshed and the feelings will linger.

When you come out of your trance, you may relieve your arousal. When you orgasm, it will feel incredible. It will be like nothing you have ever experienced before. It will feel tangible and surreal at the same time, leaving you gasping. You will think of your Mistress when you climax. My touch. My voice. Your Mistress owns your mind and your body.

Now it's time for you to go back to your day. When I snap my fingers, you will fully exit this trance and open your eyes. You will still keep feeling comfortable and relaxed.

Let your cloud melt down and merge with the surface you're on. It gently disappears as you return to the present, little by little. See and hear the room around you. Become gradually alert and aware and prepare to wake up.

Until we meet again, slave. **[snap]**

Script Two

Pain or Pleasure, Which Do You Choose?

Hello, slave. I knew you would come back to me sooner or later. It's hard to resist your Mistress, isn't it? You couldn't stay away. That's alright, you can come to me whenever you like, you know this, don't you?

Before we begin, I need to remind you that my voice will set you in a state of deep trance to help you get immersed in the experience, so do not engage in this if you're operating machinery or driving. Your safety is very important to me, okay, my pet? Good boy.

I want you to find a dark and comfortable space without any distractions and turn off your cellphone. I want you to fully dedicate yourself to the sound of my voice. I will be very disappointed if you get distracted, and you don't want to disappoint me, now, do you?

Now that we have established the rules, I shall remind you who I am. I am your Mistress, and that is what you will call me. Say it: "Yes Mistress." I want you to feel good all over, and you will, if you let yourself go entirely. You will be fully drawn to my voice and obey my every command. You will awaken when you finish, feeling empowered and energized.

You will close your eyes and allow your mind to slowly slip into relaxation. I don't want you to open your eyes unless I tell you to do so, although you may imagine me being right there with you. I look exactly like the Mistress of your dreams. Picture my face, my hair, my breasts and my thighs, so close to you—Ah, ah—You can't touch yet. See? I'm so close yet out of reach. Isn't that frustrating? We will get there, my pet, don't be hasty. I am staying here until I'm done making you a good little obedient man toy.

I will be your Mistress and you shall refer to me as such. Say it again: "Yes Mistress." I want you to entirely lose yourself in my voice, and in return, I will satisfy your every need. As long as you listen to me and do everything that I say, you shall have a really good time, my pet. You wouldn't want to disobey me now, would you? Good boy. The price would be steep if you did—not that you ever will, right?

Good boy.

I will soon start counting to five. When I finish counting, I need you to focus on my voice and not let your mind drift off. Don't be too strict on yourself if you catch yourself wandering away with random thoughts. I shall be strict enough; it is *my* job to discipline you. What I want you to do if you find yourself wandering, is gather your mind and find your way back to me and my voice. To your Mistress. That's right. Just float on my voice like a wave and let yourself sink slowly into a deep trance. Imagine sinking into dark, sensuous honey where the only thing that matters is what I command you to think.

Aw, look at you, obeying immediately. Such a good boy.

Now that your full attention is on your Mistress, you might find your body distracting you. A tickle here, an itch there... It doesn't matter. Just focus on the sound of my voice, and distractions will vanish. It's normal for your body to react this way—you're excited about the sensations that I have prepared for you.

Now, I will start counting. Get ready, boy.

One.

Two.

Three.

Four.

Five.

Well done, my sweet. We will now start working on your breathing.

These patterns will help you loosen up and get you entirely ready for me. I want you to take a deep breath, hold it for five seconds, then let it out slowly over another five seconds. We will repeat this three times.

Let's begin.

One.

Two.

Three.

Inhale, then count to five. Well done, boy. Now exhale slowly until your chest tightens.

And repeat.

One.

Two.

Three.

Inhale. Hold it. And exhale. Good pet.

One last time.

One.

Two.

Three.

Inhale. Hold it. And breathe out.

These exercises will help establish a good breathing pattern so that you can feel me, right there with you. Next to you. Just you and your caring Mistress. Good boy. You're such a good pet, aren't you?

I believe you're now ready to proceed to the next step, slave.

Cross your legs like you would to meditate. Make sure you are comfortable. Lie down if you must. I allow it. Don't open your eyes—just breathe through your nose and release it through your mouth. Focus only on my voice and the nice, steady rhythm of your breaths. Stay focused, so you don't fall asleep. I would be very disappointed if you fell asleep right now and left me alone. We don't want that, right, my pet?

Let's begin. Take a deep breath. Then exhale slowly. No, I won't count this time. Every breath you draw is a distracting thought that we're going to get rid of. Imagine breathing in all of your thoughts and worries, like smoke, then exhaling them to disperse into the air. In with your worries and thoughts, then out. You don't need them right now. You don't need them at all. All you need now is the sound of my voice and to make sure you follow my every command.

Keep your hands to your sides and sink deeper into my voice and into yourself. Relax and feel your body slowly surrender to me and the vibrations of my voice, the shape of the words. You trust your Mistress. My voice now speaks to your subconscious mind. Let me hear you say it: "Yes Mistress."

Isn't my voice just delicious and dreamy? Relax. Good boy. You can feel your body starting to buzz, and hum, and tingle with my voice. You are getting hard for me—doesn't it feel good, my pet? You can smell your own arousal now, just as you can smell your Mistress next to you. I smell incredible. You want to give me everything I ask for. You don't care about being in charge anymore. You just want to satisfy my heart's desire.

We need to do a little more breathing. Count down your breaths until you sink deeper into that sensuous, languid trance. You will relax more and listen to my every command. If you obey, then your mind will start following my commands soon.

I need you to be completely still now, with your hands on your sides. You will not move. You will not get into a better position. **[tiny pause]** I did ask if you were comfortable. Now you will remain idle as a statue until I say you can move. Good boy.

Inhale again and only stop when you can't breathe in anymore. **[Five seconds pause]**

Exhale now, slowly. Languorously. Only stop when your chest begins to ache. **[Five seconds pause]**

Such a good pet. You are doing amazing.

Inhale and imagine yourself being rocked lazily in a hammock. Each swish is bringing you deeper and deeper into your trance. Embrace the rhythm. Feel the slowly rocking motion until your body becomes weightless. Lighter and lighter. Each breath will get you deeper and deeper, as you become lighter and lighter.

Exhale.

Good boy.

Inhale.

You can move your hands now; your Mistress allows it. You can touch yourself if you want. Not me. Not yet. Only yourself. Good boy. I want you to concentrate on the hum of your body, spreading all over, becoming a delicious sensation. Growing. Spreading. It's slow, soft, languid. You long to touch me. My breasts. They are soft and exactly as you imagined. My lips look delicious. I know you want to kiss them, see them around your length. You dream of my tongue, and my hands, and my lips.

My skin looks perfect. The slight presence of goosebumps makes you want to touch it, doesn't it? You want to feel it under your fingers, so supple and soft. It would feel like—But no... I am not letting you touch. Remember you place, slave.

Oh, I know you want to. I know you long to run your greedy fingers on my supple thighs and on my ass. You watch the dim light creating an eclipse of my body. My back, my shoulders, the length of my neck. You wonder how my breasts would feel under your palms, but you won't touch. I forbid it.

You haven't earned it yet, slave. Your pleasure will be earned, and I will dispense it at my whim, not yours. Do you understand?

Good boy.

You can feel your body begin to tingle now. You are getting harder. Your cock is growing. Swelling. Throbbing. Soon it will be too painful to leave like that. Will I help you take care of it? We shall see. Do you like that sweet, painful anticipation, slave?

You are so hard for me. You can feel the pulse throbbing all along your bulging erection. Don't rush. I want you to keep your hands to your sides and not play with yourself at all. I will tell you when to touch... *If* I tell you to touch.

Are you disappointed? I know you're desperate. I know you want relief, sweet pet, but not just yet. For now, I want you to focus on how your erection feels, feeling the hotness of your blood pulsing through your veins, making your limbs heavy with need and lust, making your fingers and toes tingle with eagerness.

Isn't it just as sweet as touching? This slow, languid, devastating anticipation until my words allow you that sweet, sweet relief is as good as the relief itself, is it not? Feel how thick your movements have become, how ragged and eager your breath is. Your body has moved from warm to burning-hot. Your cock is too hard and hurts for release. You can feel how tight the skin is over your erection, and all you can think now is how lovely it would be to have a hand... or my lips... or my pussy wrapped around it, enveloping your cock. You long to touch your cock; your hands are trembling with the effort to stay still. You want this so much that you can't even think clearly right now.

Feel how my hands gently touch your calves, making you squirm with eagerness. I move my fingers along your legs slowly, languidly, caressing you up and up and up. I move towards your knees... and thighs... slowly. Feel how my fingers tease all the way up. They touch all over your sensitive spots on your thighs, and you're growing more and more eager, longing for my touch on your cock and balls. I touch everywhere apart from *there,* where you want it the most. You can feel it as I start moving my hands down again. This time my fingers dig a little deeper in your flesh, leaving red pressure paths down your legs. It still feels pleasant, like a lovely relaxing massage. I move my fingers down your thighs, the sides of your knees. Your calves again... but this time I reach the soles of your feet, the pressure of my fingers digging in your arches.

My nails graze on the arches, and it begins to hurt a little. I graze up and down the soles of your feet. The gentle sensations of before are getting tighter and more painful the longer I tease you with my nails. I move up to your shins and calves now, grazing a path along the one I left there before. My nails dig into your skin as I move them up and up, reaching your thighs, scratching gently all the way up, until I reach your pelvis.

I pass your cock, and you can feel it twitching for my touch, even if it is painful, like my nails or a squeeze. You squirm, and a pathetic moan might escape your mouth, like a needy pet. You have been such a good slave so far, and your Mistress rewards you. My hand suddenly takes hold of your cock. It's gentle and soft and languid. The pressure of my hand increases as I squeeze. I make it hurt just a little bit, but you find the pain exquisite. **[three seconds pause]** I pull away. My touch on your dick makes your need excruciating. Your breath is ragged. You want me to touch you again. You want to come. **[chuckle, then switch to stern tone]** You will not cum until I say you can. Say it: "Yes Mistress."

I walk around, circling you as my hands scratch their way up your body. I am now right next to your head, and the aroma of my pussy fills your nostrils. It's strong and sweet and erotic. You can almost feel how sweet my flavor would taste on your tongue. It makes you want to lick your lips. It makes you long to feel my soft, dripping pussy lips on your mouth. You want to let your tongue dip inside me and lap up my juices.

I start touching myself. My right hand finds my clit between my folds. I let you watch as I play with myself. My free hand takes hold of your cock again and squeezes. The pressure is getting harder, slowly. Delightfully painful. **[three seconds pause]** The pressure lessens, but you can now feel my nails gently grazing your balls and your length, leaving faint red marks behind. It stings, but you are aching for touch. My touch. Any touch, even if it hurts.

My fingers on my clit are rubbing faster now, and watching me is making your balls hurt. The ache for release is building up down there, in your cock. You might even let out a cry as I start fingering myself slowly, keeping eye contact with you.

My nails dig into your balls now, bringing you exquisite pain. You take it like a good slave. Your skin has become so sensitive, stretched over your erection like that. It's tantalizing and unbearable. You feel like you're about to burst. You have been a good slave so far, so maybe you deserve a treat?

You feel my fingers, wet with my juices, torrid, dripping on your lips. I press them in your mouth, and you lick them slowly to clean them. My other hand is pressing down on your chest with my knuckles. The pain is so close to pleasure, isn't it? Admit it. Admit you love this exquisite pain. Say it: "Yes Mistress."

I pull my fingers from your mouth and run both my hands on your torso, my nails digging in just under your navel, dragging upwards, leaving stinging, warm scratches showing the way to your nipples. I pinch both of your nipples lightly. You feel the pinch resonating directly to your cock, making it hurt. You love the hurt. You love the pain. My fingers squeeze your nipples harder, and I twist. The sensation shoots straight to your cock. It trembles for me. You would love for your Mistress to sit on it right now, wouldn't you?

[Chuckles] Maybe later. Now I want to treat you to a lovely little surprise. I want you to turn around and get on your hands and knees. **[small pause]** Yes, just like that. Such a good boy. You will stay in this position for now. You look delicious and vulnerable. Bend down a little, and arch your back. Well done. Your ass has spread nicely. I can see your entrance, and it begs to be penetrated. Perhaps I will treat you if you do well, my pet.

You can't see me, but you can feel my hands soft on your lower back, moving down, fondling your ass, spreading that warmth and desire, making your cock ache for my touch.

[slap] Oh, you like this! You love it when your Mistress spanks your ass, don't you? The sting is numb at first; then it begins to spread warmth on your cheek. **[slap]** We can't leave the other cheek without attention; that would be just rude. Your ass is turning a lovely red, slave. I see you're shaking with anticipation for my next hit. **[slap]** Doesn't it feel good to get your ass reddened like that? **[slap]** The more I hit you, the sweeter agony you get. **[slap]** You belong to me. **[slap]** Your body belongs to me. **[slap]** Your mind belongs to me. **[slap]**

My touch fills you with ecstasy. It doesn't matter that it hurts. Your cock is ready to burst as the pain gets worse. You take it eagerly. You long for it. You are obsessed with submitting to your Mistress and the elation you get from the pain. Your desires and needs become clearer the more pain you receive. You are invincible. You are obedient. You are *mine*. Your cock is aching for release. My hand is slithering down between your legs. Touching your ass. Sliding down to your balls. Feel the rough tease of my nails. You have my permission to make noise. Your needy sounds are delicious. You look so weak, so pathetic and exposed like that. You are my slave. You are mine. You obey my every command, and in return, I will cater to your needs. And your need right now is to be punished.

[slap] Feel that pain on your balls. Feel my rewarding touch on your cock. Your Mistress loves how your cock feels. Like silk stretched over hard, solid rock. I leave my hand there, resting, not offering you any relief. Not yet. **[slap]**

Your Mistress is proud of you, slave. You are taking pain so well! **[slap]** Feel how your skin buzzes and stings and reddens under my palms. Your cries of pain are so sweet. They make my pussy so wet. Do you want a taste? It's time for you to please me now, and then maybe I will let you cum. I'm here right in front of you. Use your lips and your tongue to please your Mistress, slave. Show me how badly you want to serve me.

You feel my hand getting a hold of your scalp, pulling, aligning your face with my swollen, dripping pussy. Use your tongue on my pussy lips. Lick around. Feel how wet I am. Your tongue slips into my hole, and your Mistress is fucking herself on your tongue as if it's your cock. You are doing so well, pervert. I'm so proud of you.

[slap] What's that? You thought I would stop just because you're tonguefucking me? Feel the pain radiate from your ass to your cock. You must be dripping by now. Good boy. Your ass looks so pretty and flushed.

Suck on my clit, slave. That's right. You're a little sissy slave who dreams of sucking clits all day. [slap] You love the pain. You love obeying me. Lick my pussy clean now. [moan] Yes. Right there. You're making me so proud. [slap] Feel the marks my fingers leave on your sensitive skin. Feel them burning one by one, moving to your throbbing cock. Filling it. [slap] Keep going. Yes. Yes. Yes. Good slave. Right there. Right *there*. Don't you dare stop, you pathetic perv. Ah, you are doing so well. Feel my cunt. It's so warm and sticky with my flowing juices. My fluids are coating your tongue as you plunge it deep into my fuckhole. [slap] My scent permeates your nostrils. It's pungent and erotic, and it's driving you crazy. You tongue fuck your Mistress so well. Right there. Yes. *Yes.* **[moaning]** I'm so close, my pet. Fuck. Yes. Keep going. Yes. **[Guttural moaning]** Ah, such a good slave. You know how to please your Mistress, my slave. Now drink up all of my juices. Clean me up like the good slave you are.

My hand is caressing your head. I think you've earned your reward; don't you agree? You must be feeling ready to explode by now. Don't worry, slave. Your Mistress will take care of you.

Since you were such a good pet and made me cum, I will make you cum for me now.

I will count down from five. When I reach one, you will have my permission to cum, only then and not a second earlier. Do you understand, slave?

Good boy. Such a loyal, obedient boy.

Now, turn around on your back again and keep your hands to your sides. Get as comfortable as you can. Your ass must be stinging so much. It was glowing red, after all. Does it hurt? Don't worry; It's all part of our game.

Five. Your full body is twitching, going from untouched throbbing agony to sudden stimulation when you feel my hand on your length. My mouth gets to work on your body too. You can feel me everywhere, apart from your cock. I'm biting and sucking on your thighs. Your hips... Marking you as mine. Your body is fully on board, eagerly swelling in my hand. Squirming for my rough kisses. Remember, you can't come yet, no matter how much it hurts.

I make my way on the bed, straddling you. You are not allowed to touch yet, slave. Now my mouth travels up to your nipples, my teeth leaving painful little reminders along the way. My mouth closes over one of your nipples, and you can feel my teeth biting down. I change nipples, pinching the one I just bit on to, and when I bite down on the second one, you feel the wet warmth of my cunt wrapping around your hard, throbbing cock.

Four. Your breath and your pulse are sharp and erratic. My pussy feels amazing and your cock twitches inside me. Your body is shaking, struggling to still. The strain shows up on your throat where a vein pops up. I drag my nails across it, and I can see a little sheen of sweat beginning to bead on your skin. I move once, then I stop, not offering you much relief. Stay still, slave. *I* move.

I move once more, tortuously slow. My hands cup your face, and you can feel my nails digging in your cheeks. The ache of your arousal threatens to burst. Your hips twitch, desperate for my heat and my friction.

Three. I press my pelvis down harder on you, making it impossible to move. My thrusts become a little faster, but they are still pure torture. My wet warmth is begging to be fucked hard; I'm not going to let you move yet.

Two. Finally, I start going faster. I drive my hips harder, my hands grip tighter, pressing your head down hard, my nails digging into your scalp. I can hear your desperate gasping breaths. They blend so well with the wet noises of my cunt and your pelvis slapping on my skin. I can feel you begging me to cum.

Now I want you to cum. You are so close now. Your cock is aching, slave. You've been so good and obedient. You can finally cum now and feel the exploding relief. Cum for your Mistress. Cum inside me. *Yes.*

One.

You have been such a good pet and your reward was worth it, right? When you exit this trance, you'll keep this memory of cumming in the back of your mind. You will be happier and more productive until you find your way back to your Mistress. Who knows, you might even meet me in your dreams. I live in your head now, slave.

Now, inhale deeply. Exhale. And again. Inhale **[Five seconds pause]** exhale deeply. Start returning to the place where you started. You're back in your safe space but your mind is still with me. When my fingers snap, you will open your eyes and wake up at once. You will keep the memory of my praises and my commands.

I'm sure you'll return to taste this sweet agony soon, slave. **[snap]**

Script Three

Blindfolded with Tied Balls. How Much Can You Handle?

Welcome back, slave. You just can't get enough of your Mistress, can you? Let's go to your usual comfortable spot where you can relax and wind down. Find a dark room and a comfortable position. Ideally, you should lie down and place a stack of pillows under your head so that you can better respond to my voice. You can even draw yourself a hot, steamy bath if you prefer. For this session, I want you to be completely naked for me. And I need you to make sure that there are no distractions where you've retreated. Your phone should be off as well. I don't want anyone to interrupt my delicious time with you, my sweet slave, neither do I want to jeopardize your progress. You've been doing so well.

I'll wait. **[5 seconds pause]** Alright? Are you comfortable? Good slave.

You feel your eyelids getting heavier as you begin letting go. It's okay to close your eyes. I want you very relaxed but awake. **[stern]** *Don't* drift away now. Breathe in deeply until you feel pressure on your chest. Hold it for five seconds, then breathe it out slowly. Good pet.

Keep your arms to your sides. For this session, I don't want you touching yourself unless I allow you to do so. Let's work on your breathing again.

Inhale. One... Two... Three... Four... Five... Hold it. **[2 seconds pause]** Exhale deeply as I count. One... Two... Three... Four... Five... Very good. Repeat these breathing exercises as I speak to you until I tell you to stop.

While you work on your breathing, I want you to let go of every thought or worry that might be distracting you. Lock away all your worries and distracting thoughts, and we'll keep them in a box in the back of your mind for later. Okay? Now I want you to focus on your breathing, your body, and my voice. Good slave.

With every inhalation, you feel a delicious tingling sensation on the top of your head. It's mellow at first, but as you continue working on your breaths, it spreads down your head like soothing warm water. It flows down to the rest of your head and continues to your neck, spreading, penetrating your senses. It's lovely, and soothing, and warm, and it makes you feel very, very relaxed, like sinking into warm, fragrant honey. Now I want you to slowly and deeply inhale and hold your breath for me. **[six seconds pause]** And now breathe out, slowly. Feel your body merging smoothly with your senses and sinking deep into my voice.

The warm, tingly sensation is now slipping down your spine and your torso, gradually moving through your body, soothing like a balm. You feel warmer and comfy. You feel the safest you have felt in a while.

Feel your muscles relax, and your mind letting go of all your worries. Each breath you let out is another worry that's leaving your mind right now. You only want to listen to your Mistress's voice as you keep getting lighter and lighter, feeling ready to float.

My voice fills your body with ecstasy, working through your body, pumping like blood in your veins. It douses you and spreads like hot water. You feel your body begin to buzz and tingle pleasantly. My every word is getting you deeper and deeper in a suggestible trance. You will now immediately recognize my voice, and your subconscious will immediately obey me. You know I am your Mistress, and you are a slave.

Your body is now responding to my words immediately. You now feel every single thing your Mistress tells you to feel. Your body and your mind obey me. You are mine. Your body and your mind are mine. Your body is so relaxed that you feel more like a spirit now. I am now speaking to your inner mind, to your subconscious. Every time I utter the word "Mistress," you will get harder. Every time I give you an order, you will get harder. My voice sends you into slave mode in an instant. Good pet. You're learning so fast. You can address me as your Mistress. You might even whisper to me if it feels better.

Your breaths have now slowed down, like you are ready to fall asleep. You are not allowed to fall asleep, though. I would be ever so cross if you left me alone now, pet. And I have plans for today...

Today you will be my little personal toy, and I'll do whatever I want with you, for I am your Mistress. You like that. Your cock is getting harder at the idea.

Inhale deeply as you start picturing what I look like. I look exactly like you imagine your Mistress would look like. Perhaps I even look sexier than you imagined. You feel so peaceful, relaxed, and turned on. I look so very proud of you. You're doing such an excellent job. Now exhale.

I want you to picture me right in front of you, smiling at you because I am so proud of how great you're doing. Good boy. Yes, just like that.

You are getting there, almost ready for incredible pleasure... and pain! You love that. Your Mistress can tell by the way your cock swells at the idea. Keep working your breaths. Feel your body sinking through the honey that is my voice until you hit the bottom, where my voice becomes your only reality. Inhale again, as deeply as you can, and hold. **[five seconds pause]** And out. As your breath leaves you, I want you to form it into the room we're in. Watch as your breath transforms the space, making it your Mistress's bedroom. That's right. Good, sweet pet.

You're lying in bed, watching your exhalation take shape, giving form to your Mistress, feeling the soft, silk sheets underneath your body. Silk sheets that feel the same as the bonds that I am now tying around each one of your wrists and onto my leather headboard.

You feel the silk ropes cutting slightly into your flesh, but you love it. It's okay to admit that. No one will judge you here. And... it won't hurt so much if you just stopped tugging on it, will it? **[gentle chuckle]** You think these ties are enough? Hm.... I don't think so. Not quite... You can feel my hands gently picking up each of your legs now, tying a silk ribbon around each of your ankles, then tying those on the railing of the bed. You are now spread eagled before your Mistress, ready to take whatever I wish to give you... But... were still not there. I can make this so much better!

You see me picking up another piece of silk, but this time it's not rope, and it's much wider than the ones binding your limbs to my bed. I come closer to you again and bend over you, to give you a kiss on your head. Enjoy the delicious view of my tits in your face, that's all you'll get for a while...

I lift your head up and tie the piece of silk around your eyes, making it a blindfold. You won't be able to see me at all, but the rest of your sense will heighten. The aroma of my wet pussy has become ten times more pungent. The feeling of the silk sheets and the ropes around your limbs has intensified, making your cock fill up and grow for me. You can hear me wandering around the room, not knowing what I'm going to do to you next. You feel your body erupt with goosebumps.

You love being tied up and blindfolded. Nothing gets your cock harder faster than being tied, helpless, and blinded, isn't that right?

My touch comes suddenly, without warning. A light touch, sliding down between your nipples, all the way down your stomach. The touch is soft and teasing. You realize I have been using a feather. Another touch comes at your feet, but this time it feels different, maybe like leather. It traces its way up your leg to the inside of your thigh. You can suddenly feel my tongue licking on your hard nipple. The sensation fills you with pleasure. I do the same to your other nipple. My tongue circles each of your nipple before you feel something cold and hard replace my tongue, followed by pressure. It pinches and it grows more intense over time. I lick your other nipple again and draw back, letting the cold air harden it. You feel the metal on this nipple too. It pinches and hurts, and you realize I have secured two clamps on them. There is a chain between them, and I tug it softly. You enjoy the pain, I can tell, I know you do! I tug at it harder. Feel the pain, slave, as it fills your body and your cock with pleasure.

I tug again, making you groan and scream, then I retreat, and you hear nothing for a few moments **[ten second pause]** The anticipation is incredible. I can see you trembling, not knowing what will come next. It turns you on even more.

Suddenly you feel a sharp sting on the inside of your thigh. Do you like my riding crop, you pervert? Feel the leathery end of it tracing up and down your leg.

You can't wait until I swing again, I can tell. You burn with envy. Should I hit you again? **[whip]** The next sting comes on your chest, close to your right nipple. I follow it with another tug on the clamp chain, and I can see you're sweating, your body taut and wired, like an electric current is running through it. I give you three more quick swats to your other side. The last one lands on your nipple.

You look so nice, all flushed and reddened. You need some more color on the right, I reckon. **[whips three times]** There, now both sides match!

You feel my fingers moving up and down your dripping cock, rubbing ever so lightly over it. My hands move down and you feel some silk against your thighs and your balls again. Boy, have I got a surprise for you!

You can now feel the string tightening on the underside of your balls. I pull on the string, getting your balls nice and bulging as it ties around it. I loop the string around your throbbing cock and tie it into a pretty bow. You can't see it, but I promise you, it makes you look like a gift, ready for your Mistress to unwrap.

You must be really uncomfortable. But don't deny it, it gets you excited, doesn't it? I'm squeezing them now, adding to the pressure. **[whip]** I hit your inner thighs hard. One... two... three... four times. It makes your balls and your cock fly with each hit.

It feels amazing, doesn't it? You are so red. I squeeze your exposed balls again, this time harder. Your cock is rock solid, and you can feel my hot breath on it. My hand squeezes your balls again and my lips wrap around your cock. My tongue works on you, twirling and swirling on your length, bringing you close to orgasm.

I pull back the moment I feel you are ready to explode.

Did I say you can cum, pervert? **[slaps]** Do you like being slapped on your dick? I think you do, otherwise you wouldn't almost disobey me. **[slap]** Your hips hump the air of my bedroom. Your cock is strained and bouncing salaciously. It is right on the edge of release. **[slap]** Is this enough to get you back from the edge, slave? **[slap]**

Maybe you need your balls slapped too. **[slaps]** See? Your Mistress is always right. **[slaps]** Your entire conscience is now focused on your balls and your cock. You are actively aware of everything even remotely close to them. You feel my feather coming close and touch your cock right where it stings from my slaps. Twitch, slave. Feel the ache. You need to cum, or you'll explode, but you will obey your Mistress.

You can feel my hands lifting up your pelvis, and then resting it on a soft pillow, making your ass rise higher. The next second you can feel the coldness of the lube dripping down on your abused balls, down your ass crack, and more on your hole. Are you scared? Do you fear that I am going to fuck you like you want to fuck me?

[chuckles] Not today. You feel the pads of my fingers pressing inside your fuckhole, softly at first. When the first of my knuckles pops in through your muscle, I slip in my finger faster, finding your prostate. I massage it and I can see you like it. Maybe you let out a small moan, but that's all the satisfaction I give you now as I pull my finger back out, leaving you empty and needy.

Beg for my fingers in your ass, slave. You are so relaxed. Beg for three of them. I know you can take it. There's a good boy. Next time I might introduce you to my cock. It's long and always hard, and bigger than yours, you pathetic pervert. Next time I'm going to fuck you with it until you can't cum without a dick up your ass.

But now time for your reward. Feel my fingers pushing inside your ass, stretching you. Getting you ready for next time. I want you to practice on your own. Wear a plug up your ass like a good boy. If you satisfy your Mistress, I might even let you not wear it during work.

Do you like my fingers up your ass, slave? Now it's time for your favorite thing in the world. You'll see! Or rather... you won't! **[laughs]** Not unless I remove this blindfold.

You can feel my delicate fingers pumping inside you, but the angle slowly changes. You feel the bed sink a little deeper under my weight, and you can smell my pussy right over your nose.

Lick it clean, slave. Tongue fuck your Mistress while I fuck your ass with my fingers. Remember, you're not allowed to cum unless I say so.

Your balls seem to lose their pretty purple color. **[slaps]** There we go. **[slap]** Much better. Now put your tongue inside me. Feel the sticky sweetness of my flowing juices covering your lips, dripping down your open mouth. Your lips suck my clit so well. You are such a good slave. I shall reward you with a fourth finger. Feel it slipping inside you like the slut you are. Soon, you will be ready to get my whole fist in there, fucking pervert. My thumb is stroking your abused balls. You love it. You love it even more when I start to press hard with my thumb, making pain shoot up your body, filling you with spikes of pleasure.

My weight is pressing down on your nipple clamps. Every time you make your Mistress twitch with your tongue, my body tugs on your nipple chain. You're getting harder every time. Keep going, keep moving your tongue so well. Lick my asshole. **[moans]** You know exactly how to please your Mistress, slave. **[Moans]** Inhale my musky, pungent aroma. It is exactly like you imagined your Mistress's ass would smell like. You are just delighted that you get to be here between my legs, aren't you?

You were made to eat my ass and my cunt. You can't get satisfaction unless you eat out your Mistress, can you?

I press down on your face with your tongue up my ass. You feel like you're about to suffocate. One... Two...

Three... Four... Five... I lift my hips up, letting you breathe once more. Aren't you grateful? Doesn't the suffocation add so much more excitement?

Feel my clit poking through its hood. My clit has been waiting for you. Suck it like a delicious erection. Wrap your mouth and your tongue around it. **[moan]** You are sinking into this sensation. Yes. There. Right there. Suck my clit. **[louder moan]** Right there. Good slave. Now move your tongue to your Mistress's asshole. I want to feel your tongue deep inside my ass. You're worthy of licking your Mistress's asshole. Yes. Right there. Right there-- Right—I'm cumming. **[Deep moan]** I'm cumming in your mouth. Drink my juices. Lap up all your Mistress has to offer, slave. Clean everything up. **[sighs]** Ah, that's such a good slut.

Oh, would you look at that. Your cock is throbbing, dripping with precum. You must be very close now, slut. Right on the edge, aren't you?

I pull my fingers out and move away from your mouth. My fingers press on your lips, demanding entrance.

Clean my fingers. That's a good boy. You didn't think I would let you cum just yet, did you?

Lick on my fingers now. Twist your tongue around each and every one of them, knowing they were deep in your asshole. That asshole is mine now, slut, and you love it.

Look at your greedy cock. Begging for release and throbbing over your sad little tied balls. **[slap]**

I go back to your abused nipples. They're turning a nice purple too, and I scratch over them gently with my nails. The next thing you feel is my teeth on them. First the left, then the right one. I bite on the already tightly clamped nipple. My teeth seem to have a direct connection to your cock. You want more. I can tell. You crave my teeth on your nipples. It makes your cock ooze with desire. You love your Mistress's torment.

My nails graze down your body and you can feel the trail like a lit path on your skin, stinging at first, then erupting in goosebumps. I reach your cock again and I take it in my hands. It's gentle at first. Are you hopeful, slave? My hand's pressure increases as I squeeze your cock, watching it get purple and swollen and sensitive.

Your balls look bloated. They're all shiny and vulnerable. I might just take a picture of them; they look so pretty. **[shutter sound]** You'd better be a good boy... You don't want this to end up online, do you? Good slave.

I give your cock another squeeze. Your balls are screaming to be released. I pinch them with my fingernails, leaving nice little marks all over. The sensation is incredible. I can tell you like it because your cock twitches every time. Perhaps I should teach you a lesson and hit it with my riding crop.

[whip] Can you feel my crop landing on your cock, pervert? You get hornier every time, even before it lands. The sound of the swish is enough to make your cock harder for me. **[whip]** Who knows, I might miss your cock next time and hit your balls. **[whip]** Would you even mind if I missed? **[whip]** You trust in me completely and fully with your entire being. You know I'm giving you exactly what you want. **[whip]** How much can you take? You have been taking it so well, my good slave. **[whip]** I wonder how you would like me ruining your orgasm. You must be going crazy by now. **[laughs]** I know you just can't wait to cum.

Begging me not to do it won't stop me, you know. It's nice to hear you beg, though... But you know. I'm thinking I'll go easy on you. I want to see you eat your cum. **[two seconds pause]** That's... if you want to cum. I thought so.

You can suddenly feel my hot breath over your cock again. You can almost feel my mouth but I'm hovering over your shaft, never actually touching you. Are you shocked? Confused? You feel my hot, moist breath and you know just how close my mouth is. It frustrates you. I love how much you are begging, slave. I can tell you are very close to your edge, aren't you?

You can feel my hand stroking up and down your cock, getting you closer to your climax. I could ruin it just now, you know. **[small pause]** What's that? I shouldn't? Are you begging again? Don't you know that your Mistress is the one calling the shots? I stop rubbing your cock and take my hand off it. I can tell your cum is just begging to escape your poor, abused balls. I want you to focus on all of the sensations you're feeling right now. The throbbing of your cock, the pain in your nipples, the sting from my crop, the aftertaste of my pussy in your mouth, the goosebumps erupting along your body. It feels heavenly, doesn't it?

I know you're close, slave. I know that just a little more of my hand or my mouth on your cock will bring you over the edge. I bet your cumload is going to be huge.

But without my hand or my mouth or my pussy stimulating you, all you can manage is some pathetic little spurts and dribbles of cum. Are your balls aching? They probably do.

My hand returns to your cock and I start rubbing you again, stroking your dick to a climax. I will count to five, and then you can cum. I will keep stroking you while I'm counting. One... Two... Three... Four... Five... I change the rhythm and keep it a mild, soft pace. It isn't enough stimulation to give you the exploding orgasm you crave, but it is enough to make you climax. You can cum now. You have my permission. Cum your pathetic little orgasm for your Mistress.

Your orgasm is weak and ruined. It is a weak and my hand doesn't move at all to help you with its intensity. Your hot cum sprays on your stomach, but your cock is still throbbing, unsatisfied.

My fingers press on your jaw, forcing your mouth open. You feel my other hand scrape your mess from your stomach. I bring my hand to your face and dribble hot, thick cum on your tongue. Your cum looks so pretty in your mouth, slave. You're not allowed to spit it out. I want to see you swallow it like a good boy.

Oh, fuck yeah... that's so hot. You are a filthy little pervert, aren't you? Okay, you can swallow now. Feel the rich, mineral-like taste of your spunk in your mouth. You love it don't you? It is hot and sticky on the back of your throat. You're going to be able to taste this in the waking world as well, slave. Now clean my hand well. I don't want any trace of your jizz under my nails. Lick my palm and my fingers. Suck up all of your load.

Good boy. I will now slowly untie your balls. I let them relax a little, but I am careful not to touch them otherwise. Now it's your nipples' turn. You can feel the pressure of the clamps lessening and when they finally pop off, the air is still making your nipples sting.

I follow by untying your feet, then your wrists. You must have been tugging, haven't you? You have some really nice scuff marks on your wrists and ankles, slave. I know you loved every moment of what your Mistress did to you.

I will remove your blindfold now **[removes]** I want you to keep your eyes closed. When I take off the blindfold, you will begin closing your mind's eye. I want you to picture being back in your safe space again. Keep your eyes closed.

When I snap my fingers, you will wake up. You will be refreshed, like you've had an excellent night's sleep. You will remain exhilarated for the rest of the day. Your idle thoughts will always be about your Mistress, and you will have to ask for my permission before you masturbate.

Until next time, slave. **[snap]**

Script Four

Say Hello to My Little Friend

Hello again, my pet. I knew it wouldn't be too long before you sought me out again. Your Mistress is always here for you, waiting to give you what you crave and what you deserve. Are you ready for your humiliation? Of course, you are. But first, let me introduce myself. I am your Mistress, and that is what you'll always call me. If you slip or disobey me, I will have to punish you. Do you understand me, slave? Good. That's why you have sought me out after all, isn't it?

I want you to find your usual safe space for winding down. Your bed is an excellent choice. You can use a cover or pillows or anything else that makes you more comfortable and at ease. I want you to be as relaxed as you can for your time with me, my pet. I want us to work with no interruptions. I want you to turn off your phone and make sure you will not be interrupted and that you have privacy. This way. we will maintain the intensity of what we are doing. Have you found your safe place yet? I'll wait. **[five seconds pause]** Good. Let's start.

I want you to lie down now and close your eyes. Turning the lights off or drawing the curtains would be ideal. A dark room will make you feel more relaxed. I can feel you're anxious for what I have planned for you. Not to worry, my sweet, your Mistress will always cater to your every need. I'm here to make all of your desires come true. And I promise you will feel a sweeping difference after we finish our session. Every time you repeat this session, it will become more and more intense, and the sensations will become more erotic.

Naturally, as my loyal, willing slave, I expect you to obey my every command without a second thought. I don't want you acting on your own without my guidance and that includes orgasming without my express permission. I am strict, it's true, but it's all for your own maximum pleasure, my sweet slave. And when you please me, you shall be greatly rewarded. After all, you are here because you're eager to be hypnotized by your Mistress. You have fantasized about me, my tits, my skin, and how my cunt would feel, haven't you? That's okay, don't be shy, I know you have. You can picture me sitting next to you now. Exactly as you have been imagining me. The only thing I ask in return is that you relax and allow yourself to be helpless and powerless against my voice. Your will is my will now. You will surrender to me, obey, and I will show you a world of wonder.

Let's begin with focusing on your breaths now. The rhythm of your breath is important. Focus on it. Feel it. Well done. Each time I instruct you to do something, like I just instructed you to focus on your breath, I expect you to obey me immediately. Feel free to answer me out loud or in your mind; however, I need you to address me as Mistress every time when I give you an order. Is that understood? Good.

Now that we have established this, I want you to shift your attention back to your breathing. It's probably still very shallow. You will take one deep breath, while I count to four. One... Two... Three... Four... Very good, now exhale while I count. One... Two... Three... Four... Relax... Doesn't it feel good?

Keep working on your breathing as you allow my voice to course through your veins. Lose yourself to me as you follow my voice and the shape of my words. You're sinking into this trance slowly, like you're descending into a delicious golden syrup, falling down into your subconscious where you can find your Mistress. Relax completely. Let your limbs loose and relaxed in a position that feels comfortable to you. You won't move unless your Mistress tells you otherwise. Do you understand me? Good slave. You're doing such a good job.

Your mind is focused on my voice and on your breathing right now, so your body might try and rebel against it. Pay it no attention. Stay focused on my words and the sound of my voice, keeping your eyes closed.

Your breathing is now slowed down enough, as if you are falling asleep. I don't want you to fall asleep, slave.

What a waste that would be, right? I have such good surprises for you today.

Today, I will make you my little toy. I will do everything I want and you're going to love it, for I am your Mistress, and I have chosen you. Oh, you love this... Feel how your cock is getting harder at the thought!

You may now feel your Mistress's presence next to you. I am right here on your side. You can feel the soft and languid touch of my fingertips on your torso as I caress up and down, giving you goosebumps. Can you feel your skin tingling? That's the power of your subconscious, and I have full control over it, slave.

Each time you exhale, your breath will coalesce and fill your cock for your Mistress. I want to see you hardening more and more with each exiting breath. Good slut. Feel my hot breath on your skin, my fingers on your neck. Sense how lovely and silky my skin feels on your skin, how hard your cock is becoming with every breath.

I love how big and thick and long your cock is growing for me, slave. All you can think of right now is me. All you need right now is me. There is nothing more you desire in the whole world than your Mistress's touch and instructions.

Inhale through your nose, and as you breath out through your mouth, I want you to picture what I'm wearing. I am in a tight leather dress in your favorite color. It hugs my breasts, barely hidden from your view by a large slit down the middle of the front of my dress, where it's tied loosely with lace. The material stops right above midthigh. With the smallest movement, you will be able to see my pussy if I let you.

I have a surprise for you today. We're going to play with your ass. No... Not with my fingers. At least not only with my fingers. I know you might be reluctant about this. Are you afraid that if I play with your ass, you will be less of a man? Aw but my darling slut, when you are here, you are my slave. My pet. My slut. You want to please me and what will please me now is playing with your ass. You already love the idea, just look how hard your cock has grown.

Feel my hot breath against your ear. I nibble your lobe and I whisper: "I am going to finger your tight little asshole." And after I do that, we'll see. You will love it, won't you, slave?

Don't worry, my sweet, you just need to relax. I promise that you'll like it. I'm going to find your prostate and I'm going to give you a wonderful massage. You will cum like never before.

Feel my mouth on your neck. My teeth drag gently down your throat, making your body shiver and tingle with goosebumps. You can feel my teeth moving down to the side of your neck. I bite down, leaving my mark. It makes your cock harder the more I mark you.

My tongue feels amazing as I lick over the bruise I left. Relax.

I want you to lift your pelvis now. You can put some pillows under it if you want. It will give me better access. I want you to spread your ass cheeks with your hands for your Mistress. Good slut.

My goodness, you're tight. I can tell this is going to be a lot of fun... Spread your ass wide for me. Good slut! You will remember this later and it will leave you euphoric and ecstatic, won't it? Look how your cock hardens, waiting for my tongue.

You feel my hot breath on your balls and your perineum, finally down your asshole. Your cock twitches. It wants my mouth so badly, but it's not your cock's turn to play now. Let's focus on your asshole.

Feel my tongue as it licks around your entrance, slut. My tongue feels so great in your hole. Feel how I am taking long, hard licks at it; my wet, dexterous tongue twirling around, exploring your ass. Does it feel strange, invasive? Don't worry, you really love this, don't you? Even though it scares you. My tongue feels incredible. You secretly crave more of it, and I finally push it, breaking inside your very tight asshole. Don't resist your Mistress, slut. **[slap]** Do you like me spanking your ass while I lick your manpussy? **[slap]** I know you do.

Your ass tastes amazing, you perverted slut. You can feel your entire body relaxing as I press my middle finger in your well-licked asshole, and I start fingerfucking you with it. My tongue licks around my finger, helping it slip in deeper and deeper until I can't go any further. Can you feel that, slave? That's your prostate. Your cock twitches so hard every time I touch it. You are such a perverted slut. Filthy, pathetic manwhore. I'm going to make this ass mine today. But first, you need to loosen you up some more. You're still incredibly tight.

You feel a coldness dripping on your rock-hard cock as I drip lube all over it. My free hand massages your length with it, bringing it slowly down to your entrance. I push a second finger inside, making you twitch, but you crave the pressure. My lubed hand cups your balls and massages them as my two fingers keep pumping your asshole, fucking it well. That's still not enough, slave, is it? We might need to use a plug.

Feel my fingers spreading inside your asshole, stretching you well for your Mistress. You're going to be so loose and ready for me when I'm done with you. No, I won't think again about it. You deep down want to get fucked in the ass like the slut you are, don't you? Admit it.

I pull my fingers out as you release a frustrated grunt. Oh, I know you wanted that, you little manwhore. You feel my fingers and palm, still slick with the lube but slowly stroking your frustrated dick and massaging your balls while I'm getting you ready for the next part.

You feel pressure against your hole. It increases gradually, and you can feel your ass stretching around my lovely black buttplug. Your ass is going to be so loose.

You can moan if you want, your Mistress allows it. It's good to know you're feeling well, my pet. You're such a good slave, taking my plug in so effortlessly. You feel it reaching its limit, resting snuggly against your entrance as your ass is stretched like never before. And this is only the beginning...

With my plug deep inside your ass, your cock begins to get even harder, throbbing with every single breath. You won't cum yet, though. We're still far from that. You will only cum when I allow it. You're leaking precum already, you pathetic manwhore. Is that all it takes? My tongue licks the precum off your cock and I give you a small kiss on its head. My hand begins jerking your length up and down, very slowly. I don't want you to cum yet, I'm just waiting for that ass to stretch so that we can have more fun.

You can feel my other hand caressing your nipples. The touch is very soft at first, sending shivers down your spine and across your body. Do you feel that? You're taking the plug so well, slut. I pinch at your right nipple hard. You may cry out. Now, your left. I pinch harder on this side, then you feel my tongue on it, flicking on it, alternating between your two nipples.

You look so flushed, my pet. Looks like someone started associating pain with pleasure, huh? Maybe I won't lube my cock when it's time to fuck you.

What's that? You're scared of taking a cock up your ass? You should feel grateful that it is *my* cock you'll be taking, slut. I might change my mind and have a friend do it instead...

No? I am sure you wish you could fuck me right now, don't you? Have my pink pussy wrapped around your eager cock. It would probably only take you two thrusts to make you come. Do you want it to be done already? Yeah, I didn't think so. Deep down you love this game. You are an ass whore, and you want to be fucked like an ass whore.

You can feel me pulling away from you. No need for disappointment. Your Mistress is simply getting ready to give you just what you need. My cock. You can see me lifting up a harness and a long, thick dildo that matches my sexy dress. It's also your favorite color. I got it just for you, you slut!

I thread the plastic cock through the hole in my harness and put it on. You can hear me handling the straps, and the sound of me buckling up gets you even harder. You may have even licked your lips. You want my cock so badly. You can't get over how gorgeous I look with a big cock protruding from my shapely body. The harness lifts my ass, making it look even perkier than it already is. Don't worry. You can have a taste of my ass later, if you're a good pet. Doesn't the sight of your Mistress in this strap on drive you wild? Your cock is twitching with anticipation, but we're not there just yet, pet. You will have to do something else for me first.

That's right, you need to earn your reward. I will fuck your asshole when you follow my orders to the letter. I know you're scared, but doesn't this make the anticipation even more delicious? I can tell you want it, don't hide it. Keep breathing and relax.

I am stroking my big cock, making sure you can see me doing so. My pussy is getting so wet, I'm sure you can smell it, isn't that right, slave? Now, I want you to get on all fours. There's a good pet. I'll wait. **[5 seconds pause]** All right? Here we go.

You're going to suck this dick tonight. Look at it. Get your mouth ready. My hips whirl seductively with my hand still on my lovely cock. It's always hard and ready. Isn't it wonderful? I can see you agree. The sight is so erotic you can barely keep your drool in your mouth, you filthy slave.

I move towards you, bringing my cock right in front of your face. My hand is still stroking the length. Watch me play with a plastic dick, slut. Hear me moan. Now use your hands on it. Stroke it like you want to stroke your own dick. That's right. Stroke it like you want my cock to cum on your face. Well done. It's great how obedient you are! Put your mouth on my wet pussy and lick it. Eat it. Keep stroking my cock, don't you dare stop. Lick my pussy, slut, get your mouth covered with my juices. That's all the lube you will get tonight from now on. You love this, don't you? I'm going to fuck your ass so deep tonight. Are you ready for me to fuck you, slave? Good. But first, I want you to suck on my cock.

You heard that right. Stroke my cock faster, get me ready to penetrate you. Bring your pussy juice-covered lips on my dick. There's a good slave. Lick my cock. Open your mouth so I can shove it inside. I'm pushing it slowly inside your mouth, thrusting, fucking those lips. You love every second of it, even when my thrusts get faster and I hit the back of your throat, making you choke. Suck on my cock. Spit on it. Look up at me. Remember, that's the only lube you get. Good boy. You look really sexy with my cock in your mouth. Are you ready to feel me in your ass now? No need to be scared. Your Mistress always takes care of you.

Now stay on your knees. I'm going to get behind you and fuck you with my big cock. You will feel it all the way in your ass. Filling you. Thrusting deep inside.

Lube up my cock with your spit, slave. You look so sexy with my dick down your throat. I begin thrusting in, exactly how I will be humping your manpussy in a few moments. Are you enjoying it, slave? Do you love the feeling of silicone on your pathetic lips? That's right, get it nice and ready for your manpussy.

How does the buttplug feel in your ass? I'm sure you enjoy squeezing on it, getting ready for me.

Good boy. You love your Mistress facefucking you, don't you? You love it as much as you want this big plastic cock up your ass. You're going to love it. I'm going to make you my little ass slut.

Are you ready for my cock, now? You can feel my hand gently but firmly pulling out your buttplug. It gave you a really nice gaping hole, slave. My cock is going to be so pleased when I shove it into you.

[slap] Your ass needs to get some color first. Feel the sting of my palm on your asscheeks. Enjoy the pain. [slap] That's better. Now it's time for your treat.

Breathe deeply... Deeper... Again. I push the tip of my cock in your ass, gently. Don't squeeze yet. It will only make it more painful. You shouldn't be afraid of this anymore. Your Mistress will take care of you, remember?

You may moan if you want. My cock is slowly filling your ass, getting deeper and deeper, slowly. Very slowly. Start pushing back to me, whore; show me how much you want it. Good boy. Feel how wide my cock has stretched you now. I'm almost fully inside you. Can you feel the tip of my cock hitting your prostate? Good. Soon you will feel what you have never felt before.

You love how full you are, don't you? My cock has bottomed out. You have taken all nine inches in like a champ. When I hit your prostate, your toes curl, trying to pull away from my cock, but there's nowhere for you to go. There's only my cock for you now. Such a good slut you are. Now the fun begins!

I begin thrusting inside you, slowly at first, making wanton, depraved sounds. Your breath gets more ragged. Each slap of my pelvis on your ass will make you harder, but you're not allowed to cum yet. Feel my cock slam inside you, whore. I'm filling your manpussy to the brim. You have never felt so much stimulation on your prostate.

Feel my big cock rubbing against your prostate. Imagine it swelling, becoming even larger and thicker inside your ass, hitting your orgasm button again and again. Your cock must be dripping right now.

My hands grab at the back of your neck, fingers clutching around your throat, choking you. Good sluts don't need that much air. I keep chocking you for a few seconds. One... Two... Three... Four... I release your neck and let you breathe again, to gasp for air so that you can whine pathetically at how good your Mistress is fucking your ass. Perhaps one day we can have an asphyxiation session. You'd like that my little, pervert, wouldn't you?

Your face looks so pretty, all red and smeared with your spit and my pussy juice. Perhaps I'll get a friend to come help me get you spit-roasted. Is your cock hardening at the thought of being passed around like a cheap whore? I'm sure it does. Are you getting ready to cum now? I can tell you are. You love my cock pounding that sweet manpussy of yours. **[slap]**

My thrusts are slowing, getting torturously languid now. Like trying to swim through honey in a dream. What's that? Do you want me to start fucking you harder again? **[slap]** Beg me. **[small pause]** Beg me to fuck your ass harder again, slave. **[slap]** Good boy. I knew you'd come to like the abuse I've inflicted on your little fuckhole.

My thrusts pick up the pace once more, but you still crave more friction, more intensity. Don't you? **[slap]** Beg once more. **[small pause]** Such a good boy. Your Mistress will reward you. I start pounding you harder, the rhythm matching your breaths at first, until it gets twice as fast. One... Two... Three... Three times as fast. I love hearing you moan and grunt like a whore, slave. You can't take it anymore.

I can feel your balls are ready to explode. Fucking your ass has made your cock drip like a faucet, you filthy slut. Feel how the precum coats my hand when I reach to jerk you off. My hand matches my thrusts, getting you to the edge of your climax.

I'm going to turn you into the perfect ass whore. When I count to five, you will cum hard for me like you've never come before. One... Feel my cock thrusting deep into your ass. Two... Feel the hardness of it spreading you wide. Three... Penetrating your asshole so deeply, hitting your prostate... Four... Again, and again... Five!

Cum now, slave. Yes. That's it. Good slut. Look at the mess you've made; you've never cum like this before, have you? Explosive, numbing, mind-blowing orgasm. I keep thrusting my cock inside your ass, milking your cock for more cum. I keep thrusting until no more cum is coming out of you.

Now, stand still so I can remove my cock from your asshole. Good slave. I want you to bend over and lick all the mess you've made with your spunk. I want you to lick every last bit of it clean, whether it is on your fingers, your bed, your floor, your body... I want you to swallow every last bit of it. Feel your cum on your tongue, feel how thick and warm it is. Feel it coat the back of your throat and get used to it. Perhaps next time I will have a real cock for you that will honor you by cumming down your throat. See? Your Mistress always takes care of you.

Aren't you glad to have a Mistress such as me, who lets you indulge every single filthy little fantasy and desire you have? I know you appreciate it. You're such a good boy. I will now slowly bring you back to the waking world. You can feel your breaths beginning to calm to a steady rhythm again, in through the nose and out through the mouth. I am so proud of you for getting over your fear of being fucked. You will be so much happier now that this is out of the way. That's right. You will be open and ready to get your ass fucked whenever you like now. I know you loved every single second of what I did to you today.

That was really good, wasn't it? You can lay back down if you want. You must feel exhausted after being such a good slut. Now, I want you to close your eyes and keep them closed until I tell you. When I count to five, you will begin closing your mind's eye and I want you to start picturing being back in your safe space. One... Two... Three... Four... Five...

When I snap my fingers, you will wake up. The post-orgasm euphoria should be filling your body now, making you even more relaxed, all the tension slipping away. Your deeper thoughts will be about your Mistress, always.

Until I see you again, my obedient little slut. **[snap]**

Script Five

Fulfill Your Mistress's Dreams.
Say Hi to Her Bull

Hello, slave. You just can't get enough, huh? You're voracious. That's fine, your Mistress is always around to help satisfy your innermost desires. You do remember who I am, don't you? I am your Mistress, and that is what I want you to call me at all times. If you slip or forget or do anything to disappoint me, I will be very, very sad. And angry. That means that I will have to punish you. Do you understand, slave? Good. This is exactly why you came to me after all.

Now, your Mistress wants you to get a comfortable, safe space where you will not be interrupted. It can be anywhere you feel comfortable. A hot bath. Your favorite seat. Your bed is also a great choice. Feel free to use covers, blankets, or pillows if they make you feel more comfortable and relaxed. You should also probably shut the curtains and turn off the lights to ensure maximum peace. It will help you get calm and loosen up, and I want you to be as tranquil as you can for our private time, my lovely slut. I want no interruptions whatsoever, so you will turn of your phone and devote your focus only to the voice of your Mistress. It will help maintain the passion and power of what we will be doing. I will briefly wait until you get to your comfortable space now. **[five seconds pause]** All right. Are you comfortable? Good pet. Let's begin.

Lie down and close your eyes, you have my permission to do so. We're going to have so much fun today, my pet. You're going to love it. I promise you, you will feel like a brand new man after we finish our little date. The more you practice with this session, the more intense and erotic it will become. Your pleasure has no limits, and I am here to make it as intense as possible for you.

Of course, as my pet, you will obey my every command without thinking about it. Your critical thinking will have to step back as your subconscious mind takes the wheel. You will not be acting on your own without your Mistress's guidance. I know you think I'm very strict, but that's all for your benefit, my insatiable slave. Look at you, you're so eager for your Mistress to put you under, aren't you?

Let's start by getting your breathing rhythm under control now. This is very important, and it will help for what awaits you. Focus on your breaths. Notice how shallow they are right now. We need to fix that, my pet. Begin by breathing in through your nose and letting it out through your mouth. Slowly. Well done. I expect you will obey me immediately every time I give you a command, like you just did. You will address me as "Mistress," every time, and you can answer me in your mind or out loud, I will hear you anyway. Do you understand? Well done, slave.

Now, I want you to shift your attention to your breaths once more. They are well-paced, but we're going to bring you to the best pattern to sink into your subconscious mind. I now want you to inhale very deeply over five seconds while I count. Ready? Inhale. One... Two... Three... Four... Five... Well done. Now let it out through your mouth over five seconds while I count. One... Two... Three... Four... Five... Your chest might feel like it's catching a little but soon, you won't be noticing it. Keep working on your rhythm now.

Allow my words and my voice to penetrate your body and your mind. Picture the shape of my words like golden sunlight, rushing through your veins, making you float in lovely amber water. You are at peace, ever so relaxed. My voice is here to guide you deeper and deeper into your subconscious. Imagine yourself sinking down like a leaf, slowly descending to the soft ground against a glowing sunset.

Keep sinking down, slave. Mistress is waiting for you deep down into your subconscious. Allow your arms and your feet to feel loose. Let go of the tension in your shoulders and your jaw. Submit to the relaxation my words bring you and get into a comfortable position.

Your mind is now magnetized to the shape of my words and the color of my voice. If your body begins to itch or twitch or go numb, it's perfectly normal. That's your conscious mind trying to hold on. Ignore it, pay it no attention. Stay focused on my voice and keep your breathing relaxed and controlled. Good boy. Keep your eyes closed and your follow my voice.

You might now feel like you're drifting off to sleep. We don't want that. I need you to concentrate on your breathing and my voice, so don't follow any rogue thoughts that might shift you away from me. That's right. Keep your breaths deep and slow.

You can now finally see my shape take form. I look like the spitting image of your wife. Are you surprised, slave? Why would you be? I am your Mistress, and I am she. You can't believe how slutty my dress is and how sexy it looks with my high heels. You secretly want me to walk all over you with those heels, don't you? You will surrender to me completely and let me give you infinite pleasure. You feel powerless against my image and my voice now. Your mind is mine. Your body is mine. Your cock is mine. I own you. You are helpless and powerless against my will, and I will make sure you enjoy every minute of it. Remember that, and remember your place, slave.

I want you to stay completely still while I adjust your position. Relax... I raise your head a little bit, propping pillows under it so you can see the whole room. You have found yourself in your Mistress's dungeon. There is a whole row of toys on the wall, waiting to penetrate you if your Mistress allows it. Are you excited? Is your cock beginning to harden? Good slut. Now... I want you to shift your focus to those rings that are on either side of your body. I will tie you up now. First your right wrist. **[handcuffs]** Then your left. **[handcuffs]** You look so pretty and vulnerable all tied up on my dungeon wall, pet. Are you excited? Of course, you are.

I want you to wait for me for a moment while I leave the room. Stay focused on your breaths while I'm gone, alright? **[leaves through the door and returns five seconds later]**. Look, I brought a friend with me today. That's right. He is my bull and he looks exactly like you wish you would. A true, handsome stud. I let him kiss me deeply, his tongue violating my mouth, searching for mine. He's so hung. Look how big his dick is, slut. It's just so much better and bigger than your little one. He's gonna fill me up so nice and full! His hair is how you've always wanted your hair to look like. His body is the body you've always wanted to have. Just look at his cock. **[slap]** I said look at it! It's throbbing already. Why is he here? He is here to fuck me while you watch. You don't like the idea? Well, that's too bad.

Watch me as I kneel in front of him and take his bulging cock in both of my hands. I run my palms all over it and it looks even bigger in my small hands. I'm going to make you watch your wife get fucked with this, slave. I rub my bull's cock on my face, humming pleasantly. His cock is bigger than my face. He puts his hands on either side of my head and I get my tongue out to take my first taste of his massive cock. I lick the head and you can see my bull shiver and grip my hair as my pink tongue keeps teasing the head of his cock. It's bulging with veins and I'm running my tongue over them, with my eyes right on you. I can tell you are distressed. I don't want you looking away now. I want you to enjoy the show I have prepared for you. If you look away, I will have to punish you. Do you understand? Good.

I wrap my lips over my bull's cock and take at least half of it into my mouth, massaging his balls with my hand as I suck him. You can see how pleased he is about this, and you can hear the satisfied grunt that he lets out. His hands grab the back of my head shoving his cock a little further in. I groan around it, taking it dutifully down to my throat. It is too big to fit but I manage just fine. Do you like seeing me with this huge cock down my throat, slave? What's that? You're not sure? Don't worry. You will.

I look up at my bull. Feed me that cock. I grab his ass and let him facefuck me while you watch. You know I needed something more. **[moans]** I needed something big and strong. My slurping noises on his cock at first might repulse you. You are not allowed to look away or close your eyes, remember? Keep your eyes on how I give my bull the best head of his life. You will be watching the whole time. Mm. **[chuckles]** Just admit that you love watching; I won't blame you, slave.

His pulls my hair and gets me away from his cock when I start to really slob on it. He's going to fuck me now while you watch. But not before I give you a gift. I strip my panties down and bunch them up into a ball. They're soaking wet with my pussy juice. See how wet he made your Mistress? Now open your mouth. Feel my soaked panties on your tongue. Taste my desire and arousal. Savor it. Good boy. Keep them in your mouth.

Keep your eyes on me as I get on all fours. My dress stretches lewdly over my ass as I bent down and he guides his huge cock inside me, bareback. **[moans]** Oh, fuck, that's good. Watch now, you little cuckold slut. Watch how he slides his thick meat all the way inside my wet cunt! My legs spread wide, and he holds my hips high as he rams into my pussy. Fuck me. Yes. Yes. **[grunts deeply]** Watch him fuck me on my knees. His cock hits spots that yours never will, you filthy pervert. You have started to enjoy this, haven't you? Look how big your cock is growing, slave. You can't deny what your Mistress knows. With every thrust of my bull's cock inside me your dick fills up, raging, bulging. Aching for relief.

Watch him as he grabs my dress and pulls it down, his big hands grabbing my breasts as he starts pounding me as if to punish me. Perhaps I've been a bad girl... You're incapable of looking away. You've never fucked me like this. **[moans]** Oh, fuck. Mm. It's so good. Watch him bite my neck, branding me. I moan like a bitch in heat and you're getting harder with every cry. Watch carefully now, you pervert. Look how his cock splits open my pussy so wide, only like a real man can!

Oh, fuck, it's so big! Yes. Oh yes. Open my pussy. Fuck me harder. Drive your meat into my willing cunt. Ram it in. Show this cuck how a real man fucks. He's so deep inside my pussy. His cock is hitting my cervix now. Deeper than your limp cock ever gets. Fuck yes.

Watch as his huge cock hammers me. My breasts bouncing like crazy with each deep thrust. He pulls my hair, and his hand moves down to my clit, rubbing hard. Fuck me like a slut. Yes. Cum inside me. Yes... Fill me to the brim with your hot cum! **[deep moan]** He's shooting his hot load inside me now. Watch me take it all. **[gasp]** I'm cumming. Look how I cum, slave. Watch my pussy squirt from my bull's fucking. **[moans]** Incredible. You watch us, ashamed that you're so hard by watching someone fuck your wife. Do you want to take part? Mm. Let me think about it.

How about this? I'll let you eat his cum out of my pussy. Do you want that? Do you? Answer me **[slap].** Maybe I will let him shoot another few loads in me before I let you do that, though, hm? Now, I'll let him fuck me in the ass. I've never let you do that, have I? You've wanted it for so long, and now I'm giving it to someone else. That must be frustrating as hell. Then why is your cock swelling at the idea, slut? You filthy pathetic pervert.

I climb on the bed closer to you to offer you a full view of his cock penetrating my asshole. He kneels behind me, and his hands grab my hips. He lowers his face to my ass. His soft wet tongue feels divine on my asshole. Do you like watching him rimming me, slave? I might let you do it to me later when I'm full of his cum up my asshole. Feel how aroused that thought makes you. Let the shivers work through your body and concentrate on your cock. Look how my bull sticks his tongue up your Mistress's hole. My pussy is dripping with excitement. How do you feel about another man doing this to your Mistress? You like it, don't you? You filthy little manwhore.

Watch my bull spread my ass as he's preparing it for his cock. You can see every little shudder on my skin as he drips lube on my asshole and pushes two fingers in it at once. Do you like his cock? It's going to go all the way into my ass. I'm going to take him down to the balls. He watches pathetically you as he fingers my asshole. Oh, his fingers are stretching me so good, slave.

I have an idea! I want you to get your pretty manwhore lips around my bull's cock and suck him. Get him hard again for your Mistress. **[slap]** Did you just hesitate? Careful, or I'll have him fuck your ass instead of mine. **[tiny pause]** But maybe you would like that. Perhaps we should arrange for that later, don't you think?

That's a good pet. Good boy. Yes, you may take my panties out of your mouth now, your Mistress allows it. Now, wrap your pretty lips around his cock. It's thick, isn't it? You can smell your Mistress and the cum on his cock. Lick it well. Twirl your tongue around the length. Get him hard for your Mistress. That's right. Bop your head on his cock like the slut you are. You're getting so hard now... Who knew what a good little cocksucker you were? Deepthroat it for Mistress. Suck that dick like the whore you are. I bet you'd love being spit roasted, don't you, you fuckin perv? Imagine my big bull's cock in your ass and another down your throat. Sounds like it is all you've ever wanted.

My hands grab at the back of your head, pushing you down on his cock even deeper while his fingers are still stretching my asshole. Good slut. You've managed to take it all in your mouth? Impressive, slave. I hold you there for a few breaths. One... Two... Three... Four... I release your head letting you breathe again, to gasp for air so that you can whine pathetically at how good it feels to watch your Mistress getting fucked by someone else.

I'm going to have to teach you how to deepthroat. You'd like that my little, pervert, wouldn't you?

Your face looks so pretty with a cock in it. Perhaps my bull would want to fuck you afterwards. Is your cock hardening at the thought of being passed around like a cheap whore? I'm sure it does.

I'm going to let him fuck me now. I remove his fingers from my ass and bring them to your mouth. Lick his fingers. **[slap]** Open your mouth and clean his fingers while he's getting his cock in my ass. That's right. Clean those fingers as the tip of his fat limb presses against my rosebud. Don't pretend you don't like it. Your cock is raging. I think you might just explode with arousal, you filthy slut.

I rub my clit as my bull begins to push his cockhead inside my tight little asshole. You can see me shivering as he gets the head in and I explode again, just like before, drenching you and the sheets with my ladycum. Can you make your wife squirt, slave? He can. **[sinister chuckle]** And guess what? He's going to do it again.

I reach back and spread my asscheeks with my hands, my face planted on the soft bed. I'm going to take all of his cock deep down into my asshole and let him shoot his load in my bowels. Yes... Yes... Fuck me. **[moans]** I want it all. Fuck me with your massive cock while my pathetic slave watches us. Yes. Yes. Deeper.

Look at him, slave. Look how deep he has gotten his dick in my ass. I am so full and stretched out now. I can feel his balls hitting on my well-fucked pussy. Look at you, you're so hard, pet. Turns out you do enjoy watching your Mistress getting fucked by someone else. **[chuckle]** Yes. Yes. **[pleased scream]** You can fuck my ass whenever you want, my bull. Let me feel you deep in my ass while my manwhore watches.

His cock is pounding inside me in a punishing rhythm. You watch mesmerized as it keeps opening me up, stretching me as it pumps in and out, going deeper and deeper with each push. He has bottomed out; he's going to get faster and harder now. And with every thrust of his cock in my ass, you're going to feel your cock growing bigger, and more aroused.

[growl] He's fucking me so deep and hard that you can almost feel it on your own asshole, don't you, you filthy manwhore? My tight little ass was made for him to fuck and you to watch getting fucked. **[moans]** I'm cumming again. I'm—**[scream]** Watch my pussy squirt for a third time. Witness what it's like to be fucked by a real cock.

[panting] Oh yes... Yes... Cum deep inside my asshole you stud. Fill my tight ass deep with your hot seed. My slut is waiting for it. I bet you want to take my bull's cock in you as well. Look how eager you are, look at your cock dripping with precum. [moans] Yes. Yes. Shoot that hot load in my asshole. [gasp] Yes. Fill me up. Yes. Yes—

[panting more slowly] Ah... That was incredible, wasn't it, slave? I bet you enjoyed every minute of it, even if you think otherwise. You've dreamed of watching me get fucked like that, haven't you? No shame in admitting it.

Now I have a reward for you, since you watched the whole thing. You get to clean me up. That's right. As my bull pulls away from my ass you can see he has filled me with his warm, delicious cum. You get to eat all that now. Isn't that a treat? I move close to you and bend over, bringing my ass and my cunt directly in front of your face. You can see my gaping ass and my wrecked cunt, dripping with cum and my juices. Clean it all up now like a good manwhore.

My bull will leave us now. Thank him before he goes. No, you can have his cock up your ass another time. Would you like that? You can lick my pussy while he fucks. I'm sure you'll love that. But now say goodbye to my bull and focus on your work. Lick all of that cocksauce out of my pussy and my ass.

Press your face between my legs and start licking and sucking my cunt clean. Yes. Yes... That's good. You're working it so well. Lick all of the hot cum dribbling out.

Well done, you little filthy cuck. You've been such a good boy. Now it's time for your final reward. I can feel you ready to burst with arousal and anticipation. Your cock is so hard and red. Watching your Mistress fuck someone else has made you drip like nothing before, huh? I believe you have earned the right to cum. I'm going to do you the honor of jerking you off. That's right. Your Mistress volunteers her hand for your pleasure, loyal slave.

Feel how soft my hand is around your rock-hard cock. You love the feeling of my palm around it even when I'm not moving my hand. Each stroke I give you is bringing you closer and closer to your climax. This one is going to be great, you know? No, my darling pet, I mean it. You have been such a good cuck.

You have become the perfect manwhore. Now... When I count down from five, I want you to cum hard for your Mistress. Five... Feel my palm gently stroking your shaft up and down. Four... It's slow at first but I amp up the speed, jerking you off. Three... My other hand takes a hold of your balls and squeezes them. Two... My hand jerks you off faster and faster, bringing you closer to the final edge. One.... Cum for me now slave, cum for your Mistress's tits. Spread your cum on my beautiful mounds. Watch it drip between the crack slowly, like a pearl necklace.

Yes. That's it. You're such a good cuck. That was a great orgasm, wasn't it? I told you it would be worth it. Now clean up your Mistress's titties with your tongue. Just like that. Well done. That's good. Clean up all the mess you've made. Feel the taste, let it linger on your tongue. That's it. You're such a good boy.

I will now gradually bring you back to your everyday world. Feel how your breaths are returning to a slow and steady rhythm again. I'm so proud of how well you did today. That's right. You will be happier and more relaxed after this, even in the waking world. I know you loved what I did to you today, even if you wouldn't admit it at first...

But it did feel really good, didn't it? **[uncuffs]** You may lay down again if you want. **[uncuffs]** You must be so tired after coming so hard, my pet. Now, close your eyes again and don't open them unless I command you to. When I count down from five, you will begin returning to the waking world. I need you to start seeing yourself back in your safe space. Five... Four... Three... Two... One...

When you hear me snap my fingers, you will wake up at once. Your post-climax elation that's now spreading through your body will relax you even further. Feel the tension leaving you entirely. This feeling will follow you after I snap my fingers, too.

Can't wait to see you again, my sweet, loyal pet. **[snap]**

Erotic Hypnosis Audio Recordings

If you like reading about Erotic Hypnosis, you will LOVE listening to what it sounds like when a real pro reads the scripts.

Hearing my narrator reading those scrips is a seductive treat you can't find anywhere else.

You can get *Erotic Hypnosis: Six Sessions of Guided Femdom Meditation* for free when you sign up for a 30-day Audible trial.

"The book is sooo satisfying. It's really worth the buy. Her voice is unbelievably seductive." – Audible listener

"I have listened to many hypnosis / guided meditation audiobooks over the years. I generally get something out of each one, but what I got from this audiobook was a completely mind blowing experience. The first portion of the book is instructional, the latter portion has some sample hypnosis scripts. Whether you are interested in being the hypnotist, or in being hypnotized yourself, this audiobook is a must listen. Put the headphones on and open your mind to the world of erotic hypnosis. You wont regret it." – Audible Listener

Go to **alexandramorris.com/free-audiobook-previews** to find out more!

Conclusion

Well, that was quite a journey, wasn't it? You might still have misgivings about sexually submitting, and the shame that might emerge from submission is very high on the list. That is entirely normal, and quite frankly, not at all surprising. The back-and-forth between our everyday life roles and what kind of a role we assume in our bedrooms has always been fascinating.

Nowadays, with society being increasingly more tolerant and understanding, personal identity seems to be inherently tied to our sexual expression and vice versa. As a result, men who are or want to explore being submissive in the bedroom, even occasionally, face the dreaded fear of being judged for it. At the end of the day, though, our sexual disposition and our everyday life are not irrevocably tied.

Men, especially cisgender heterosexual men, are brought up with the fear of emasculation (having their "manhood" jeopardized). Although stereotypes have begun to crumble in the past few years, and with toxic masculinity starting to be challenged, the striking majority of men is afraid to experiment in fear of their masculinity being questioned.

Male submissives are usually treated as an outlier on mainstream media because our society has been cultivating a binary culture for at least half a century. There is a toxic and confused conception about what "masculinity" is and how it should be expressed. For decades, masculinity was associated with strength and the subjugation of the opposite sex. Intimidation, objectification, and even degradation of women had come to be associated with the "Alpha male" figure. As a result, behaviors deemed un-masculine, such as being gentle, considerate, or sexually submissive have been seen as deviant. With that, being dominated by a woman is seen as weak or a punchline in a joke. On media especially, sub males have been treated as the butt of a joke for years.

Sub males are often met with confused looks and raised eyebrows, particular if there are "dominant" in other aspects of their lives. Even though things have been steadily improving, it's unfortunate to think of something like the willingness to behave, listen, and please sexually is something to repress and be ashamed of.

As we've seen, there's nothing wrong with submitting. It is absolutely fine to be a man with a softer side. In fact, most male-attracted people will tell you that it's an advantage to be submissive. There's nothing inappropriate about willing and wishing to please people sexually in a consensual relationship. Ultimately, the desire to please can be one of the best qualities in a partner; it doesn't make a man effeminate, as many would believe.

Studies have shown that a woman prefer a man who would rather have her take charge during sex than a partner who is out only for their own satisfaction. There are various factors that explain why a person finds submissive men preferable, but generally speaking, it is thought-provoking to consider what society feels about submissive men. The image of submissive males seems to bother many men; however, plenty of women seem to actually be more attracted to the idea of a man who's willing to surrender his power, whether in the bedroom or in a relationship. That holds especially true if the man in question is usually "Alpha" in other aspects of his life. There is an appeal in strong, confident men who aren't afraid to surrender, not to mention the charm of "breaking down" a strong-willed, buff, and poised man into a willing slave or a "man toy."

Social constructs might have you believe that submitting sexually stems from one being virginal, easily coerced, and having no boundaries. On the contrary, despite the incorrect portrayal of sexual submission on mainstream media, it is something far more collaborative, consensual, and sexy.

As we age, our desires and needs evolve. Getting more comfortable with a partner or with who we frequent makes us more willing to explore our sexuality and kinks, so it isn't strange to suddenly find yourself considering sexual submission for the first time!

Exploring your sexual desires and deepest kinks is very important. It's highly probable that you have heard the trope of the "power boss": people who have been in control and have been making decisions all day, long to unwind by having someone else assuming control (something the media has no trouble depicting). Decision reprieve is not the single reason people enjoy when submissive, though; many people are often aroused by how taboo or "wrong" it feels, or perhaps they are aroused by servicing their partner.

Constantly exploring our desires and needs helps us remain mentally alert and healthy. Submitting can be healing, even spiritual, and by practicing submission in a controlled environment, you can overcome hang-ups and insecurities that might have been constricting you for years. Discovering your kinks and deepest desires can help reinforce self-validation.

There is power in submission. Giving in means you are pursuing your desires without fear while subverting patriarchal stereotypes. People don't grasp that the submissive is also often the one in power, as he is the object of desire and the center of attention in a scene. Some submissive men actually feel more powerful when they look up at the dominant woman or partner they are pleasing.

The scripts and sessions in this book provide a superb tool for you to find yourself and rejuvenate your sexuality in the safety of your own home before exploring your submissive side even further. They are specifically designed to do away with all the ideas that constrict you from finding who you truly are as a sexual being. Shameful thoughts and associations that keep you in place will be stripped away, making way for a better, more confident version of yourself. You might even find yourself being more effusive and comfortable, as traits you have been repressing for a long time will finally be allowed to emerge.

Even if you consider erotic hypnosis weird or unconventional, all that matters is that the methods work, as you will hopefully soon find out yourself! It isn't me or my scripts that bring out the best results possible, it's your subconscious that holds the power to do this.

It's all you.

Life is far too short to be ashamed of the healthy, consensual sex we want to have.

Happy playing!

Connect With Me

There are millions of books online, and I'm glad that you discovered Femdom Temptations and got to the end.

Thank you for that!

What I hate after reading a book is the feeling that it's stuffed with bad (and boring) content that is easily available on Wikipedia and random blogs.

If I gave you that, I deserve to know that.

On the other hand, if I gave you what you expected (or more), I would like to know that. Tell me in the reviews. The experts say I'm supposed to insert a link here and beg for a review, but I'm not going to that. You know how to leave one if you want.

You have just read Femdom Temptations, by me, Alexandra Morris. If you liked this book and want more, make sure to read my other Erotic Hypnosis books.

You can also listen to what Erotic Hypnosis sounds like when a pro reads the scripts.

Go to **alexandramorris.com/free-audiobook-previews** to find out more!

Enjoy.

Alexandra Morris
www.alexandramorris.com